Steps in Rhyme

Bath Time

Written and illustrated
by Courtney Katos

Light Muse Studio, LLC

Dedicated to my mom,

who always made sure I had books and art supplies.

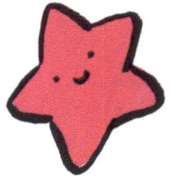
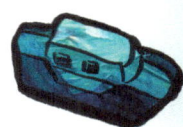

Light Muse Studio, LLC
Copyright ©2025 Courtney Katos.
Illustrations copyright ©2025 Courtney Katos.
All rights reserved. No part of this book may be reproduced or transmitted in any form or by any means, electronic or mechanical, including photocopying, recording, or by any information storage and retrieval system, without written permission from the author. The final page of steps may be photocopied to post for personal use.

The author is not a trained therapist or doctor, but rather a mom/teacher/artist/author hoping to help someone. This book is for informational purposes only and is not intended to diagnose, treat, or replace consultation with a licensed professional. The publisher and author make no guarantees of success following the content of this book, and your use of this book implies your acceptance of this disclaimer.

For information contact lightmusestudio@gmail.com.

ISBN 979-8-9922082-3-8
10 9 8 7 6 5 4 3 2 1

To my dear readers,

Everyone learns in different ways, and many people prefer when learning is fun. This book teaches the steps of bathing with rhymes and bright pictures. So have fun with this book and get yourself clean!

To the parents, guardians, teachers, and caregivers,

As a parent and educator myself, I find that many kids learn better when I set directions to a little rhythm or rhyme. I also know how helpful it is to repeat instructions often as I teach a skill. I hope this book of rhyming sequences and textural visuals will make the process easier and more fun for both of you.

At the end of the book is a small version of each illustrated step. You may copy this for your personal use if you would like to post it in the bathroom as a reminder for your child. You could even cut out each image separately for them to arrange in the correct order.

Happy reading and happy teaching!

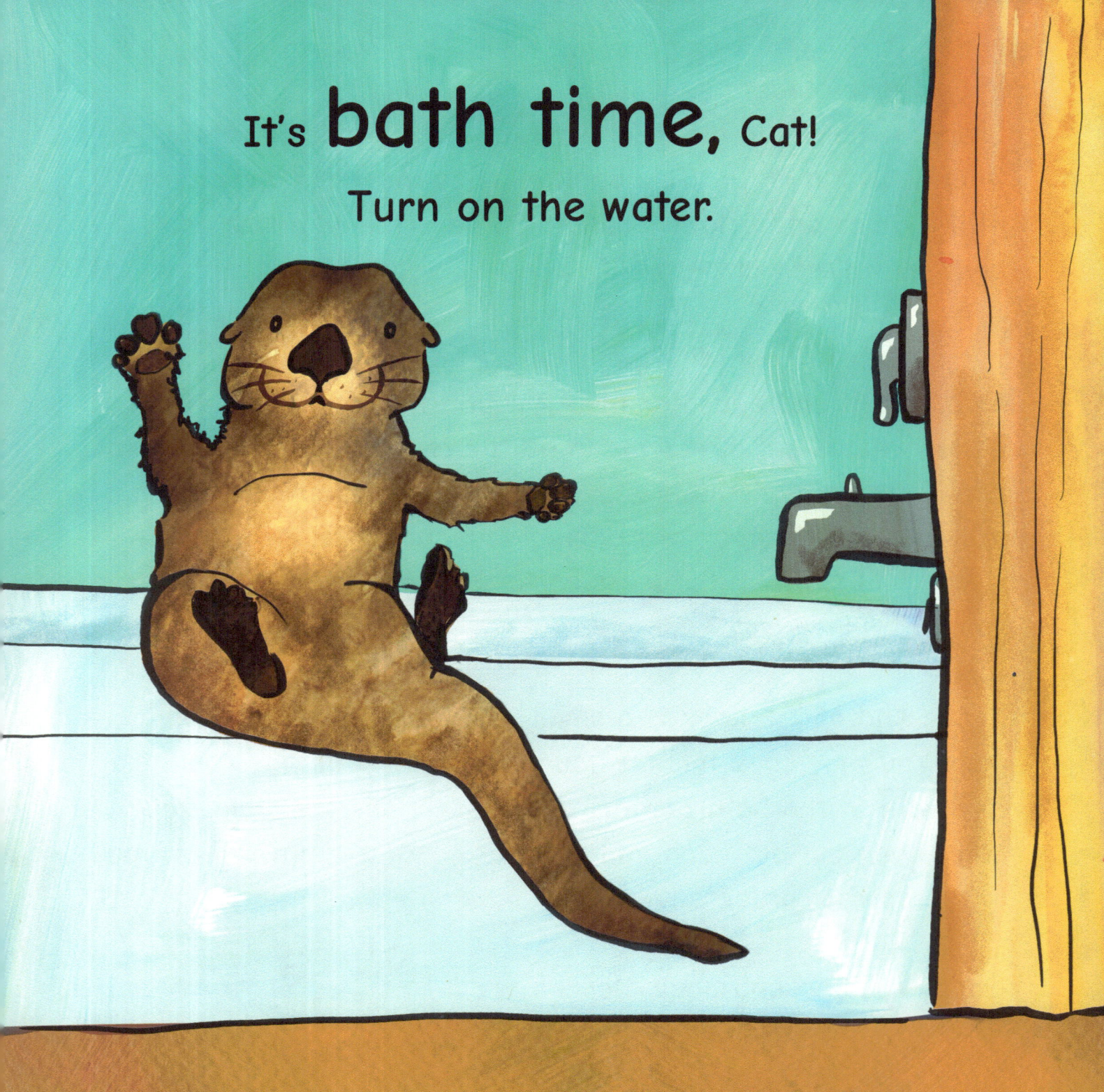

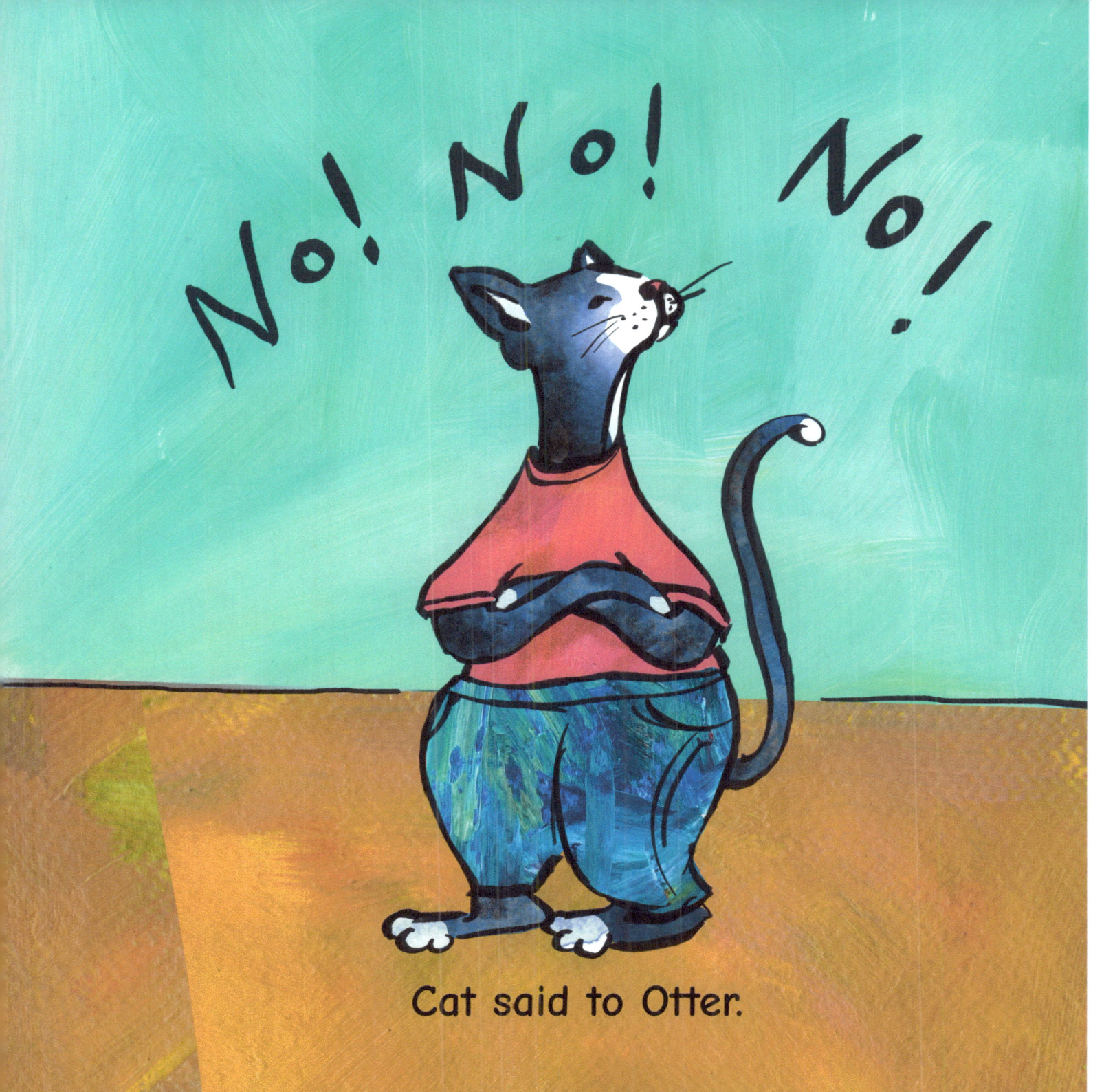

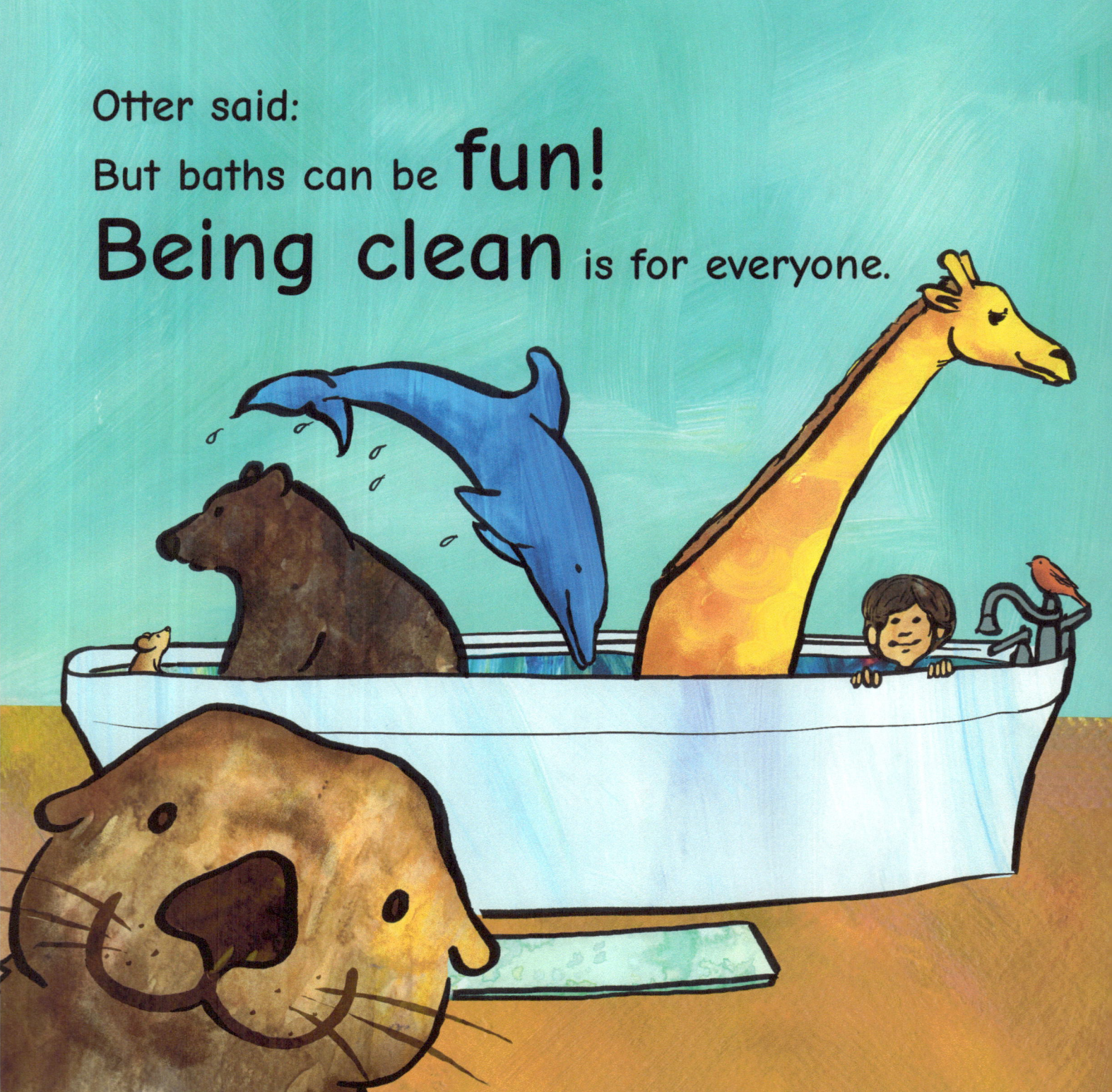

Otter said:
But baths can be **fun!**
Being clean is for everyone.

First make sure your grown up knows,

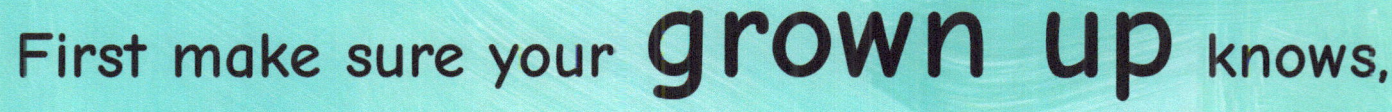

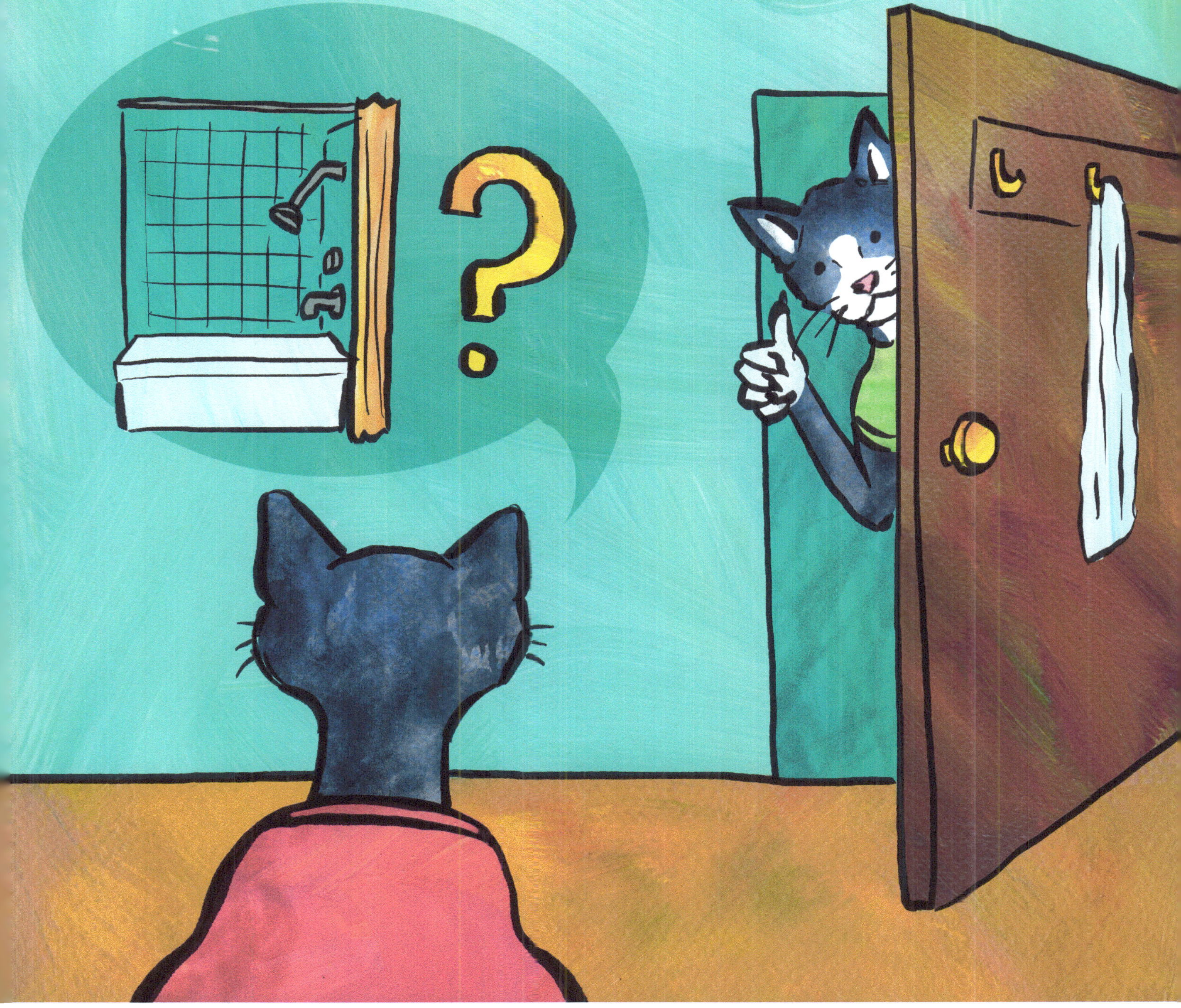

then take off all of your clothes.

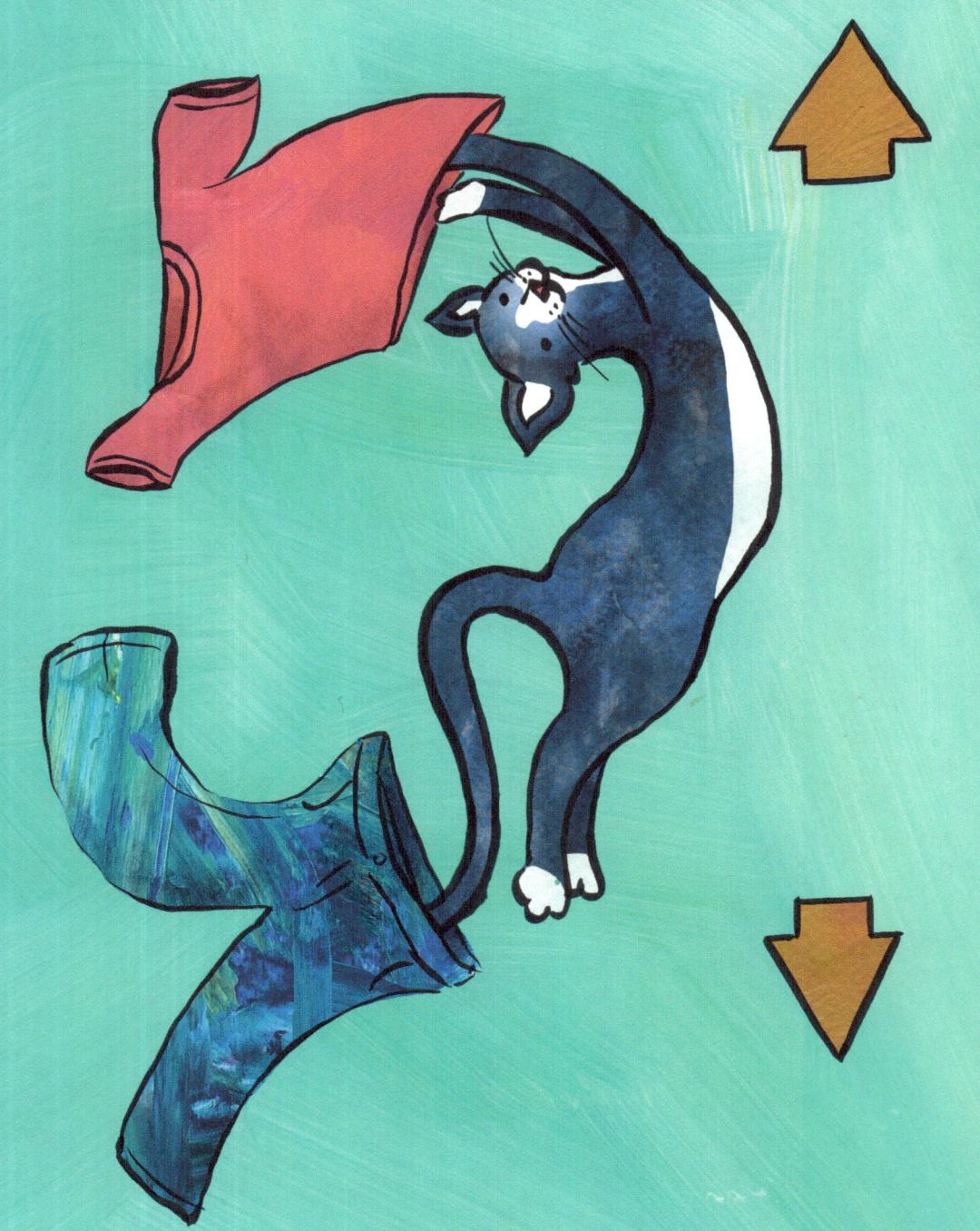

Make the water **warm** to begin.
Not too hot or you'll hurt your skin.

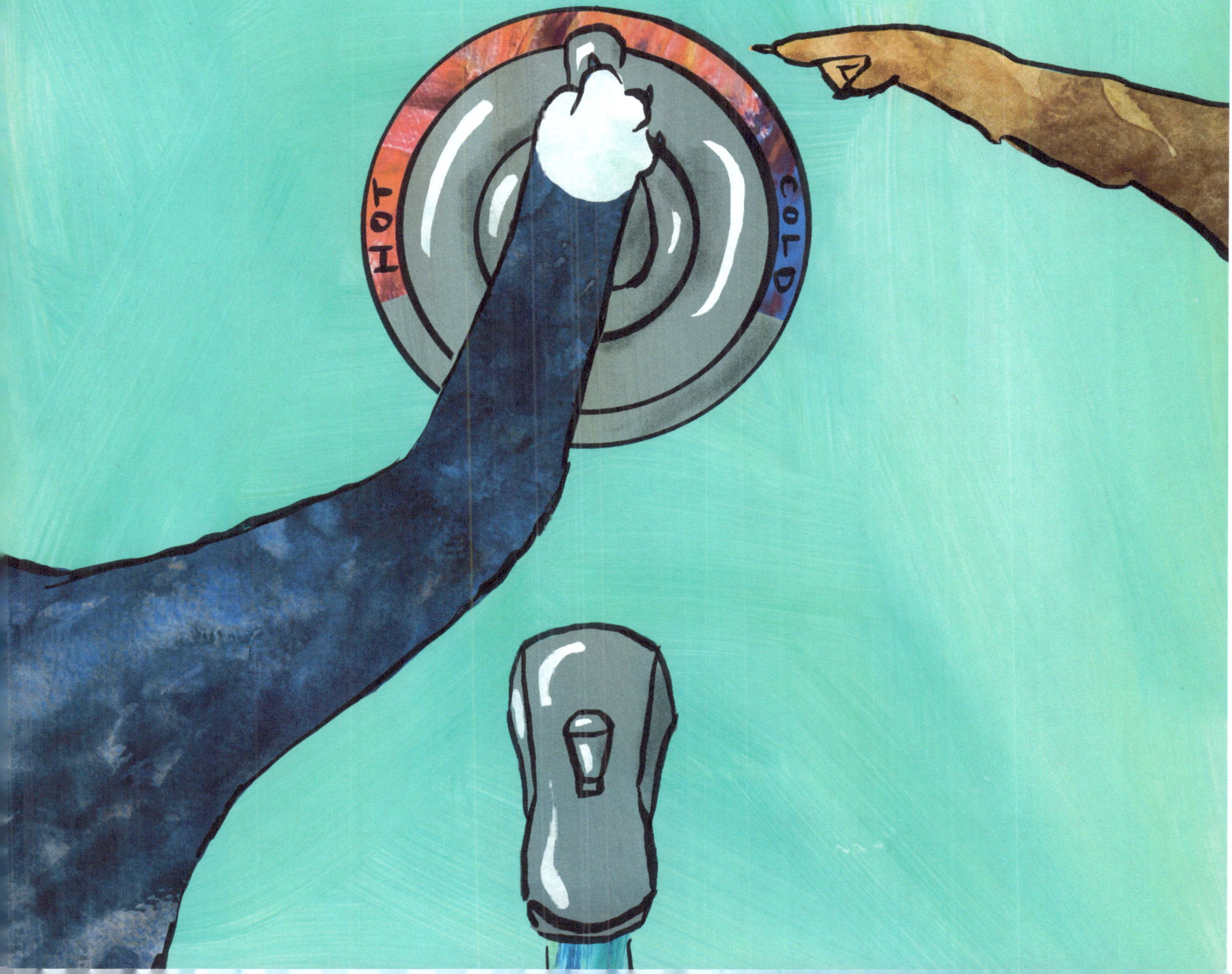

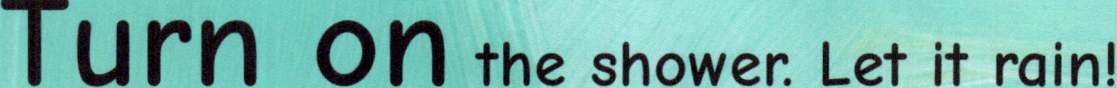
Turn on the shower. Let it rain!

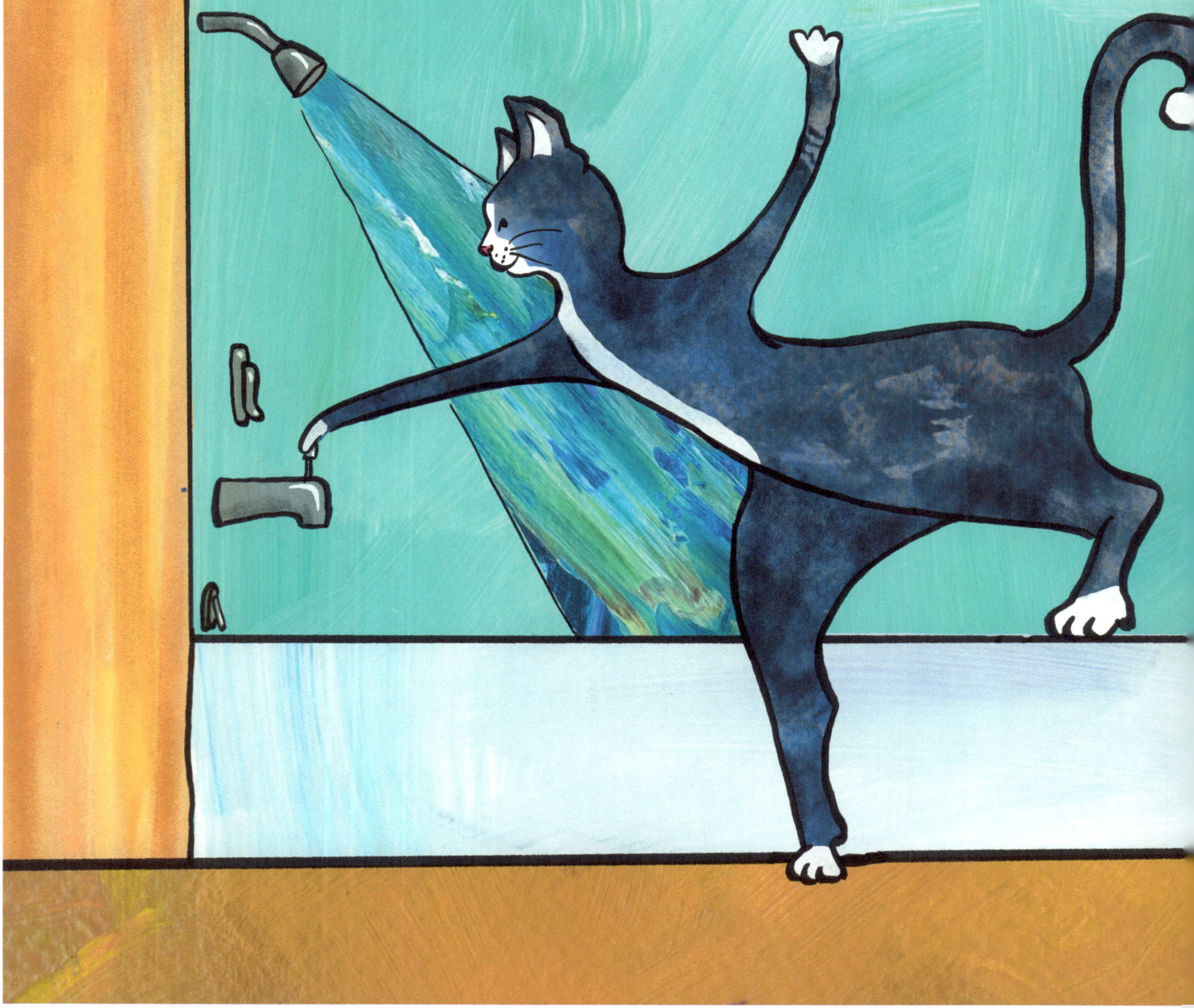

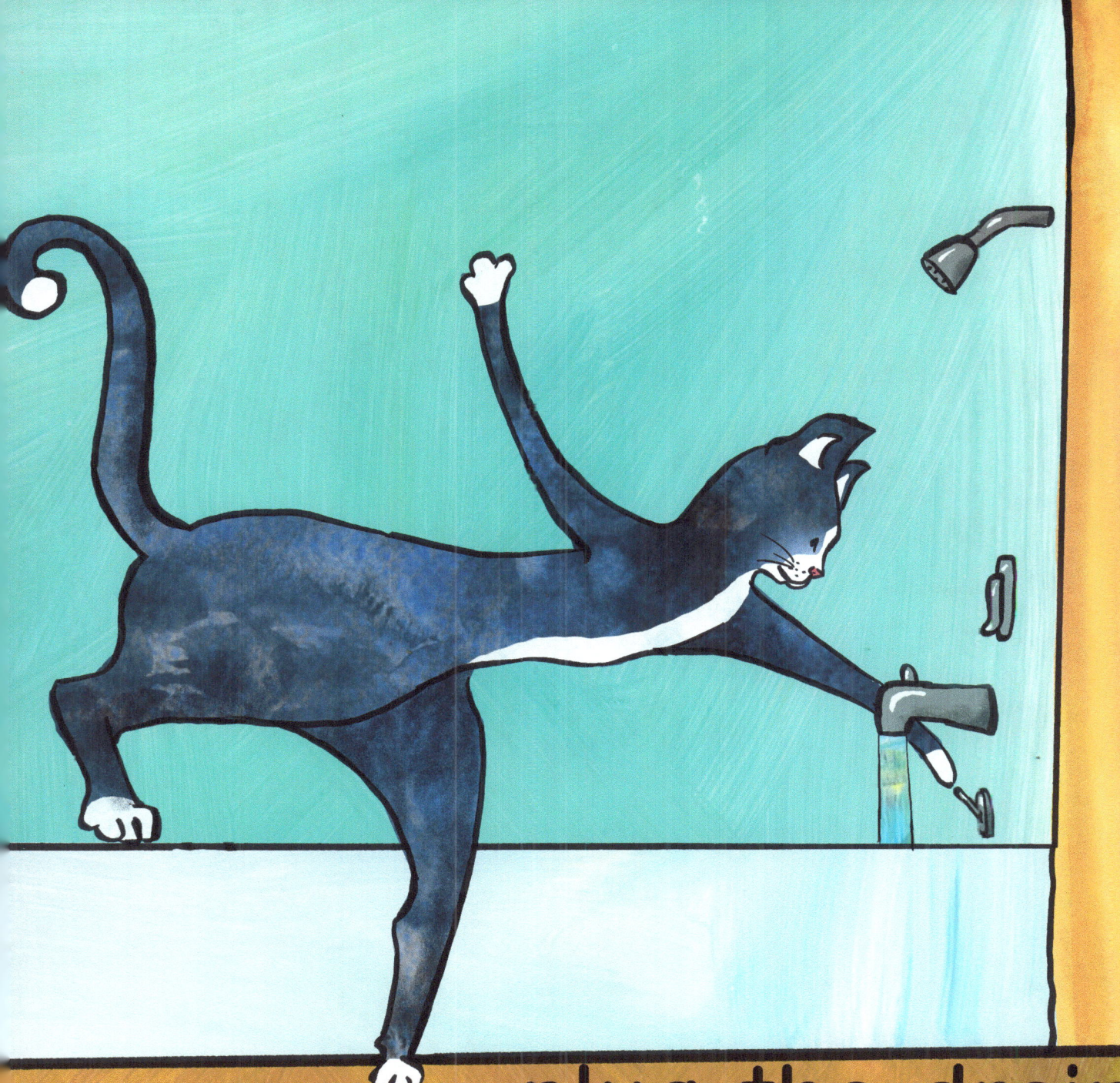
Or for a bath, just **plug the drain.**

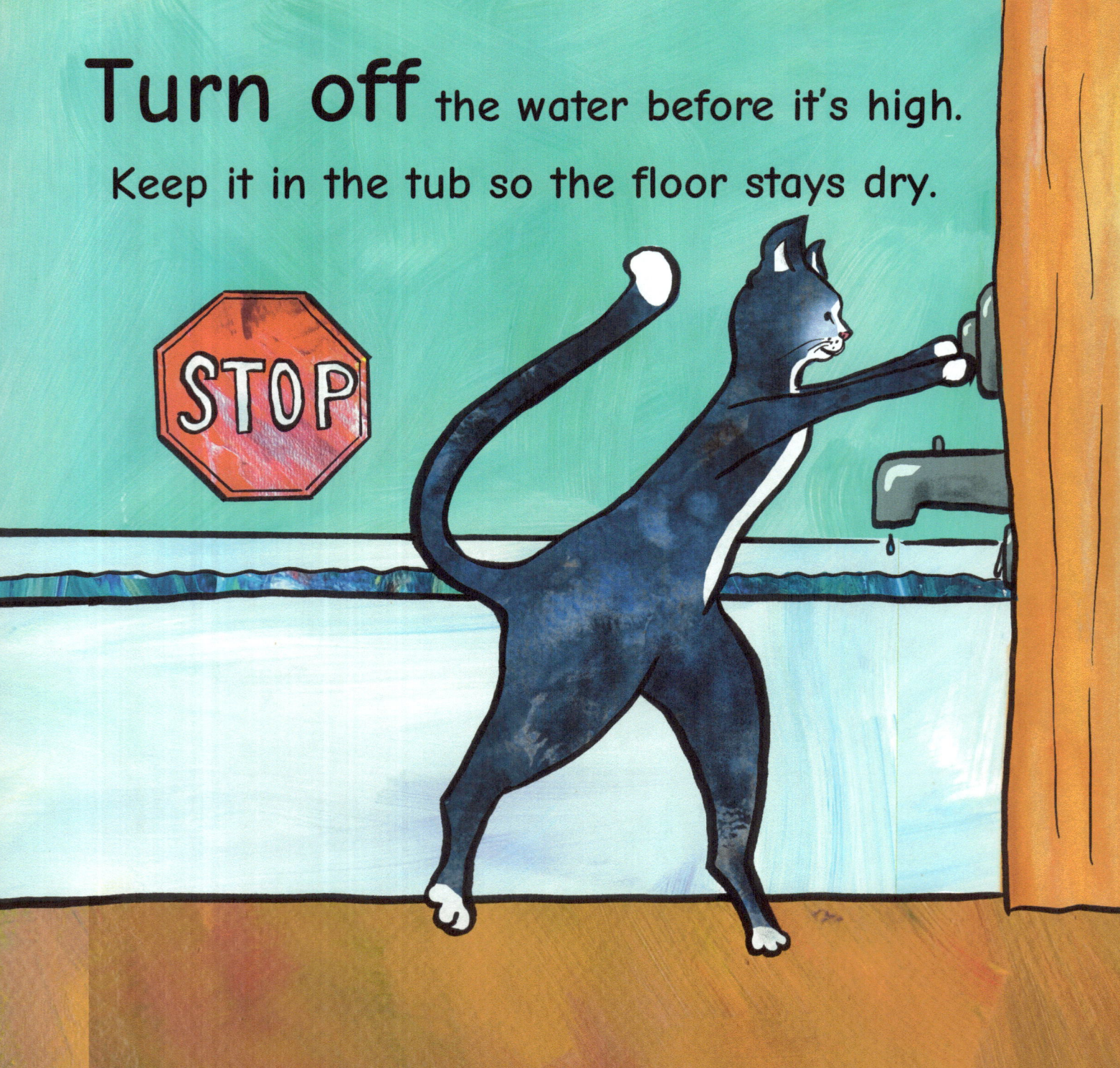

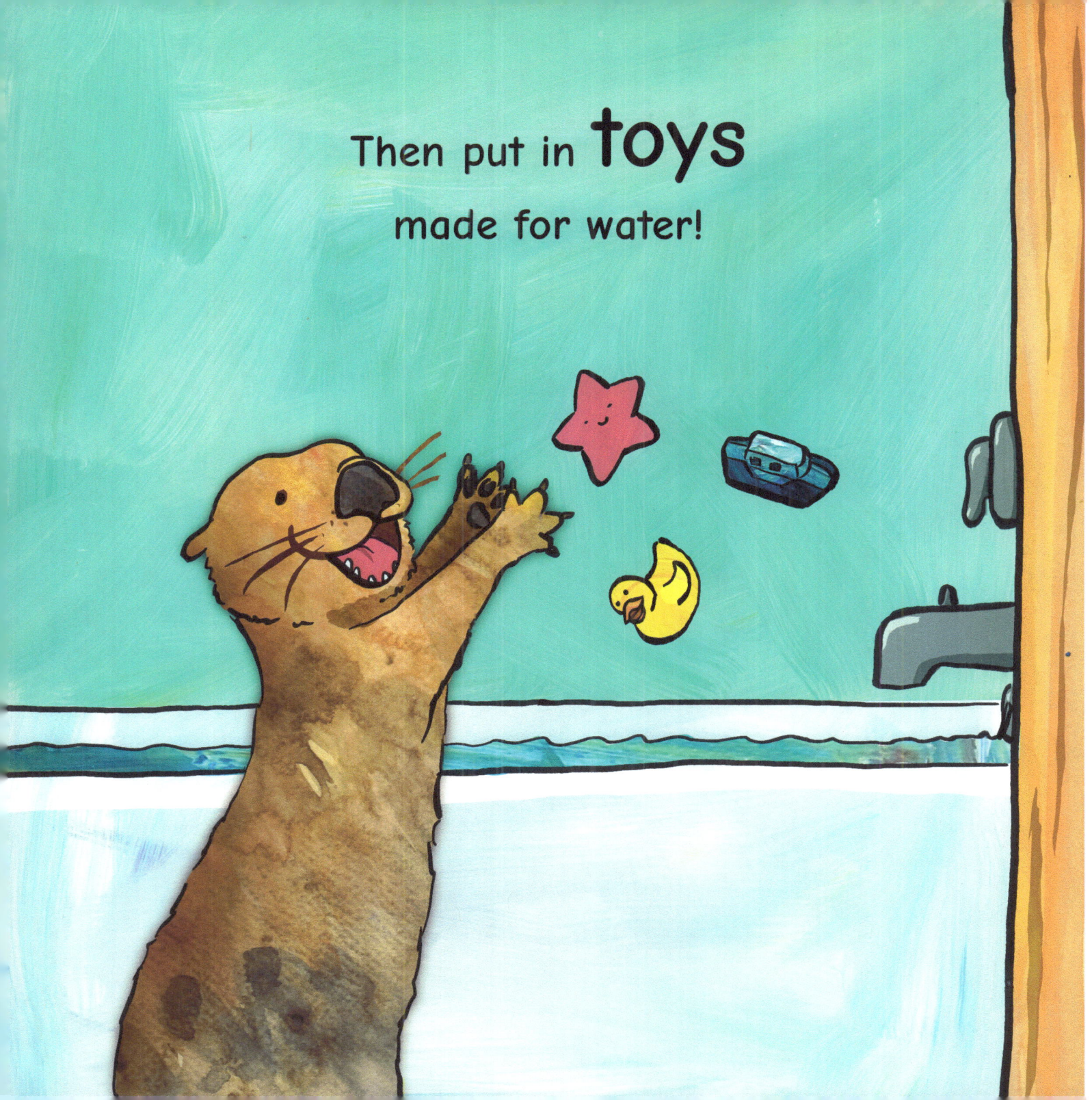

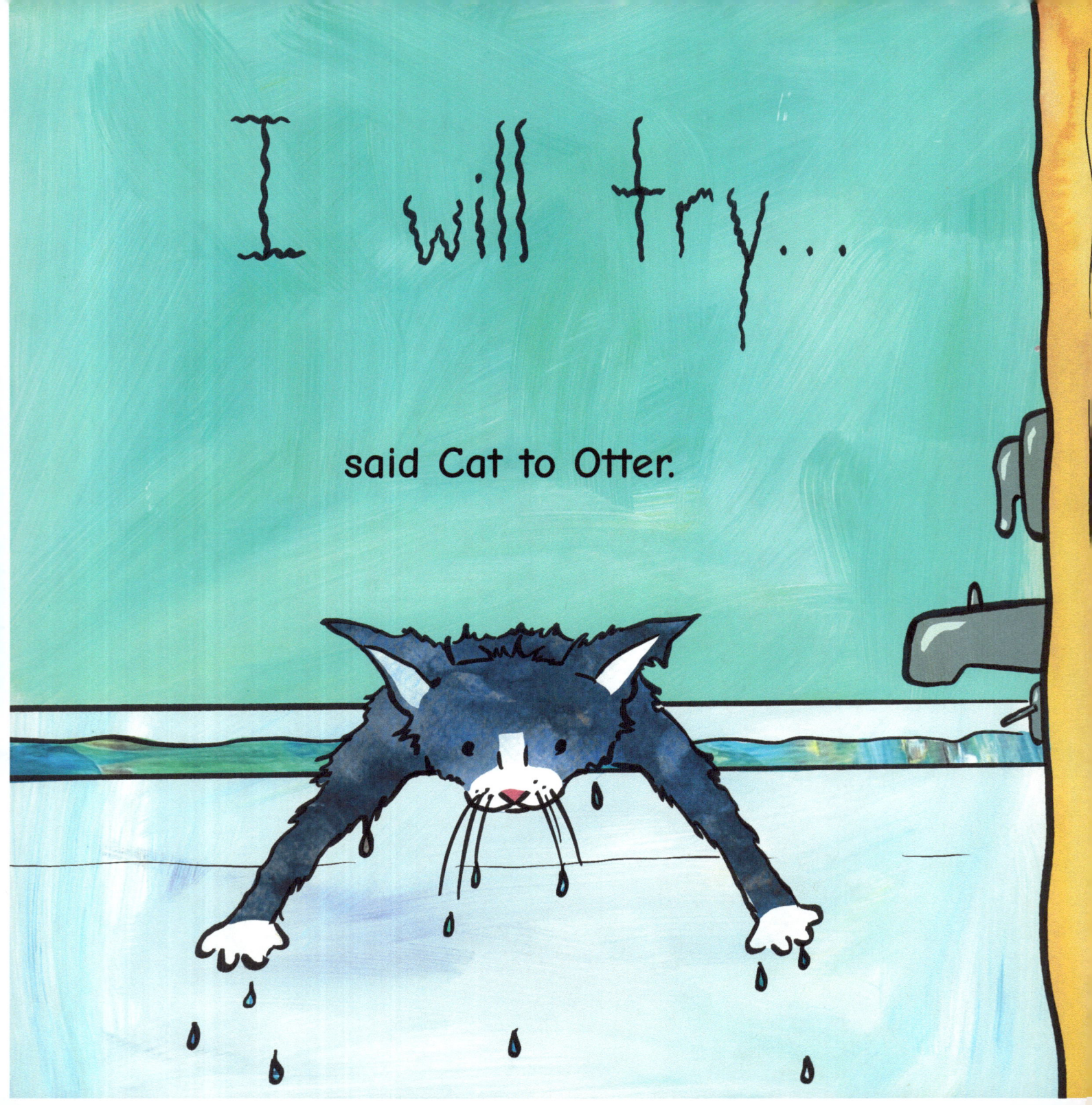

Once you're wet, squeeze out

shampoo.

A little

on your hair

will do.

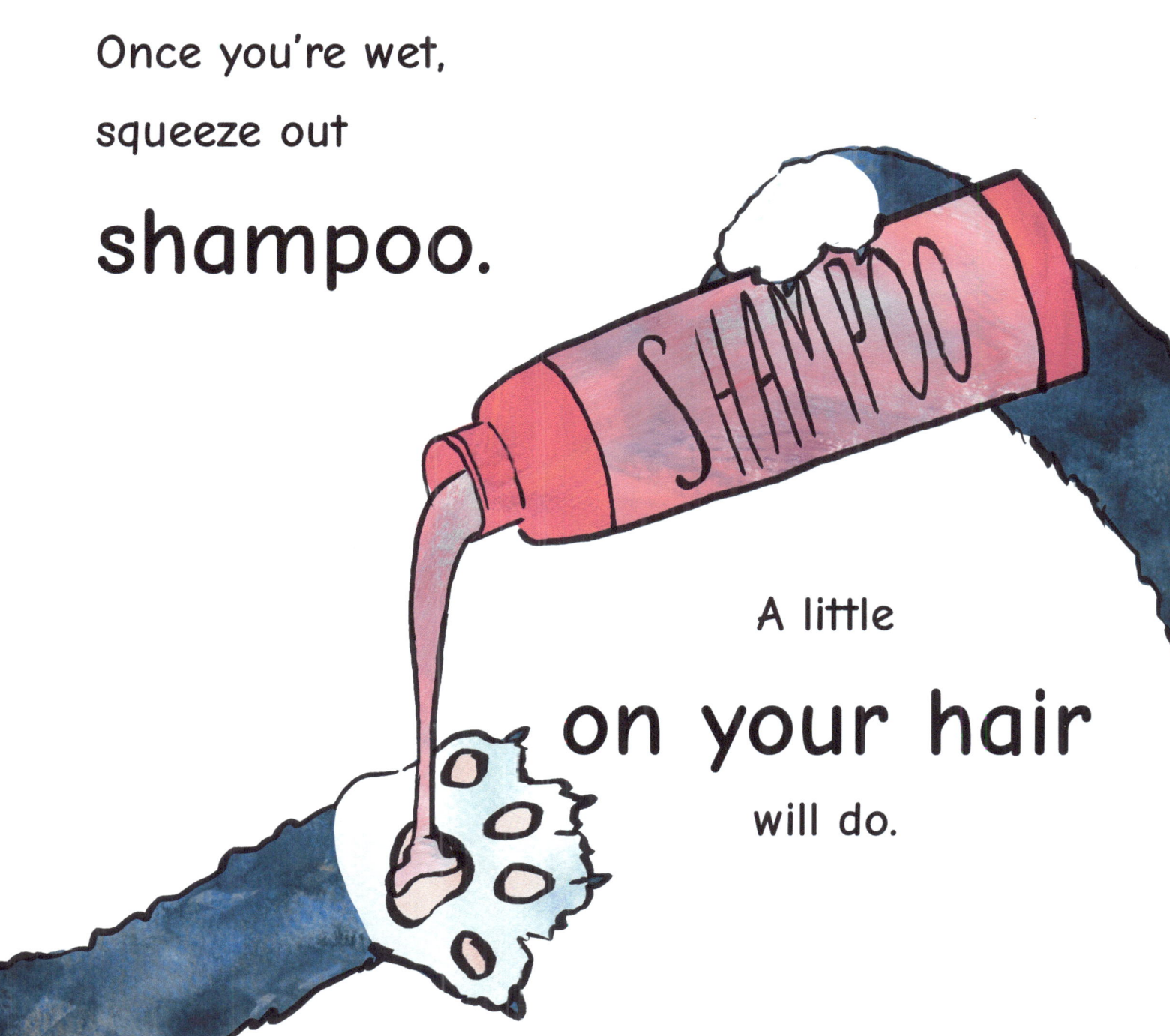

Rub, rub, rub

to make it bubble.

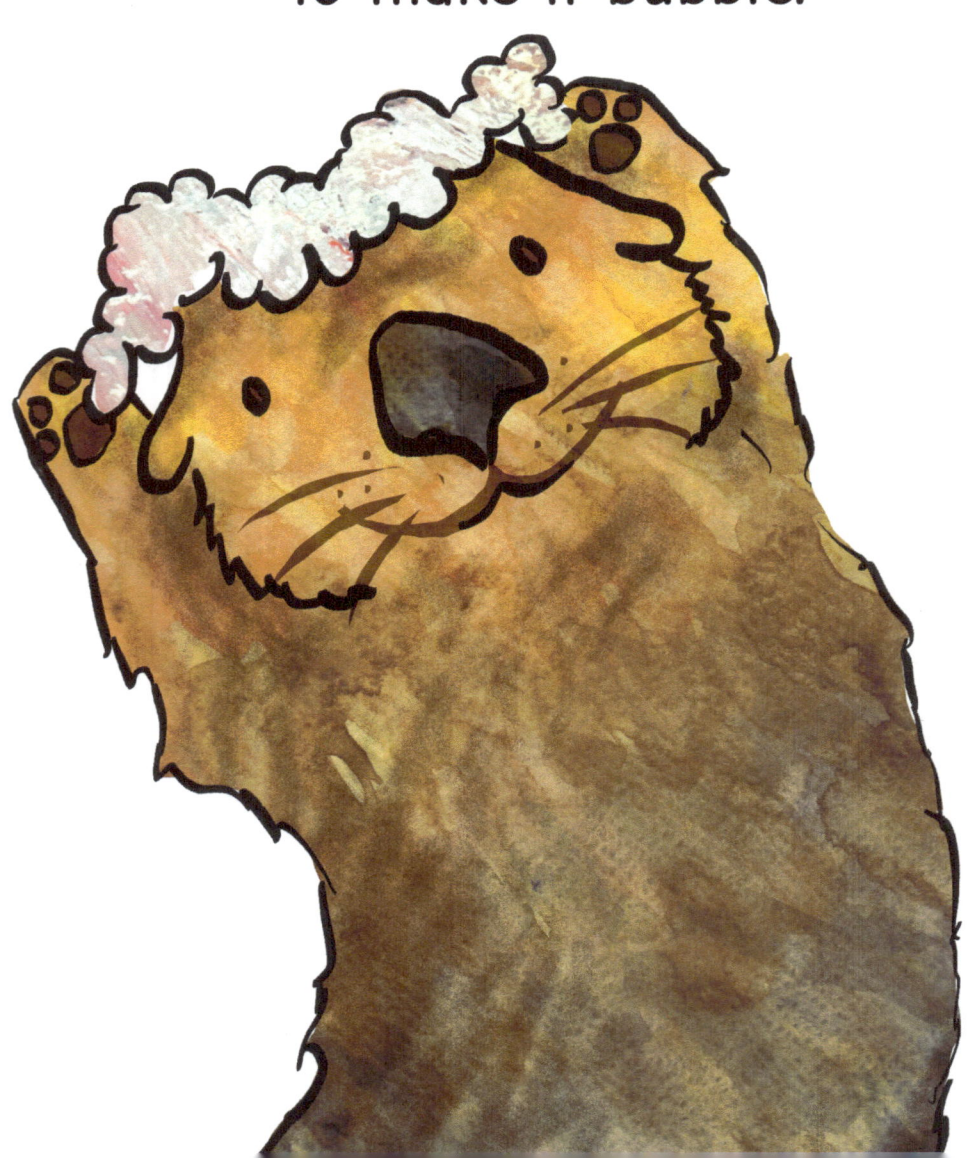

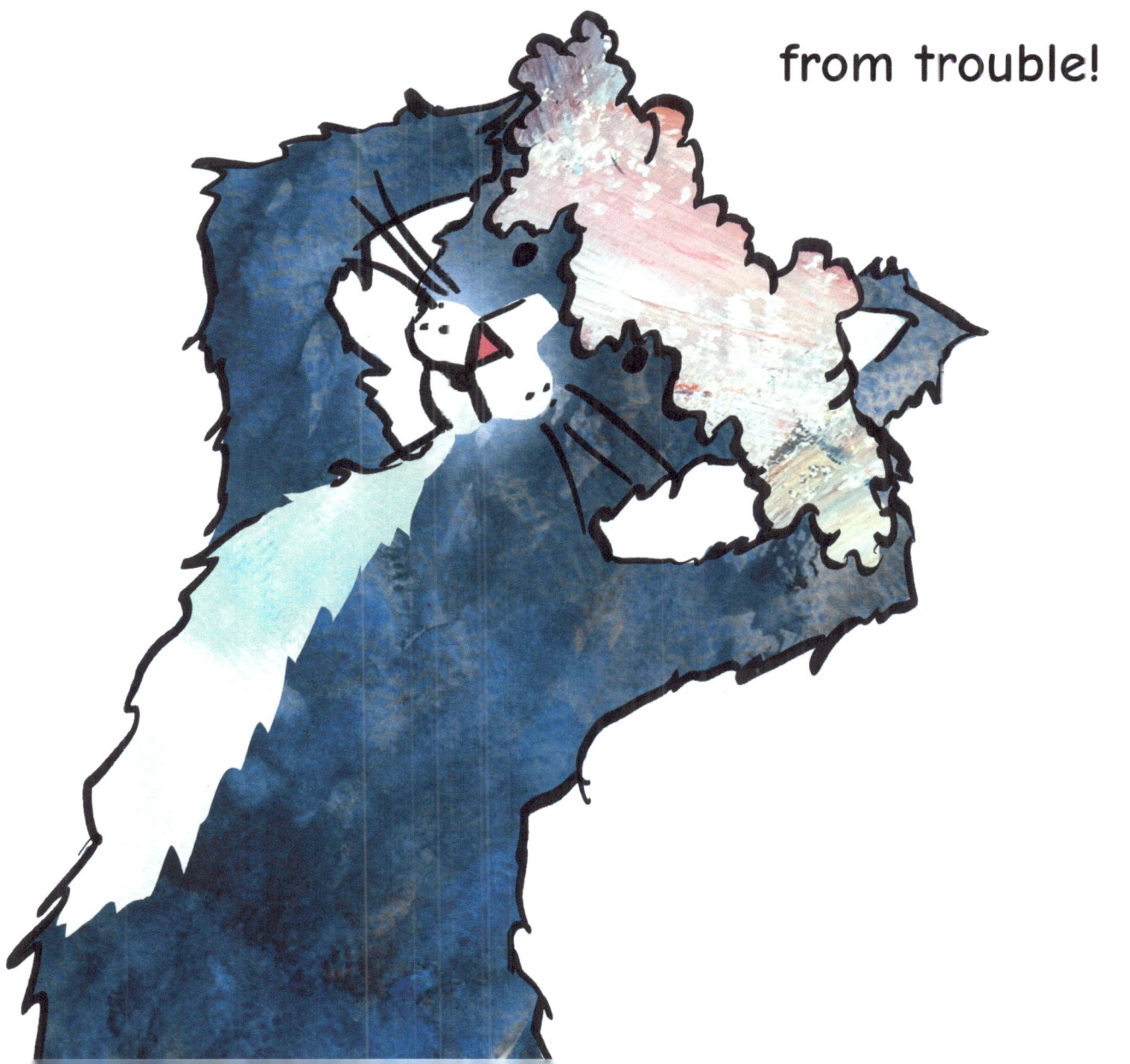

Cover with a cloth when you rinse,

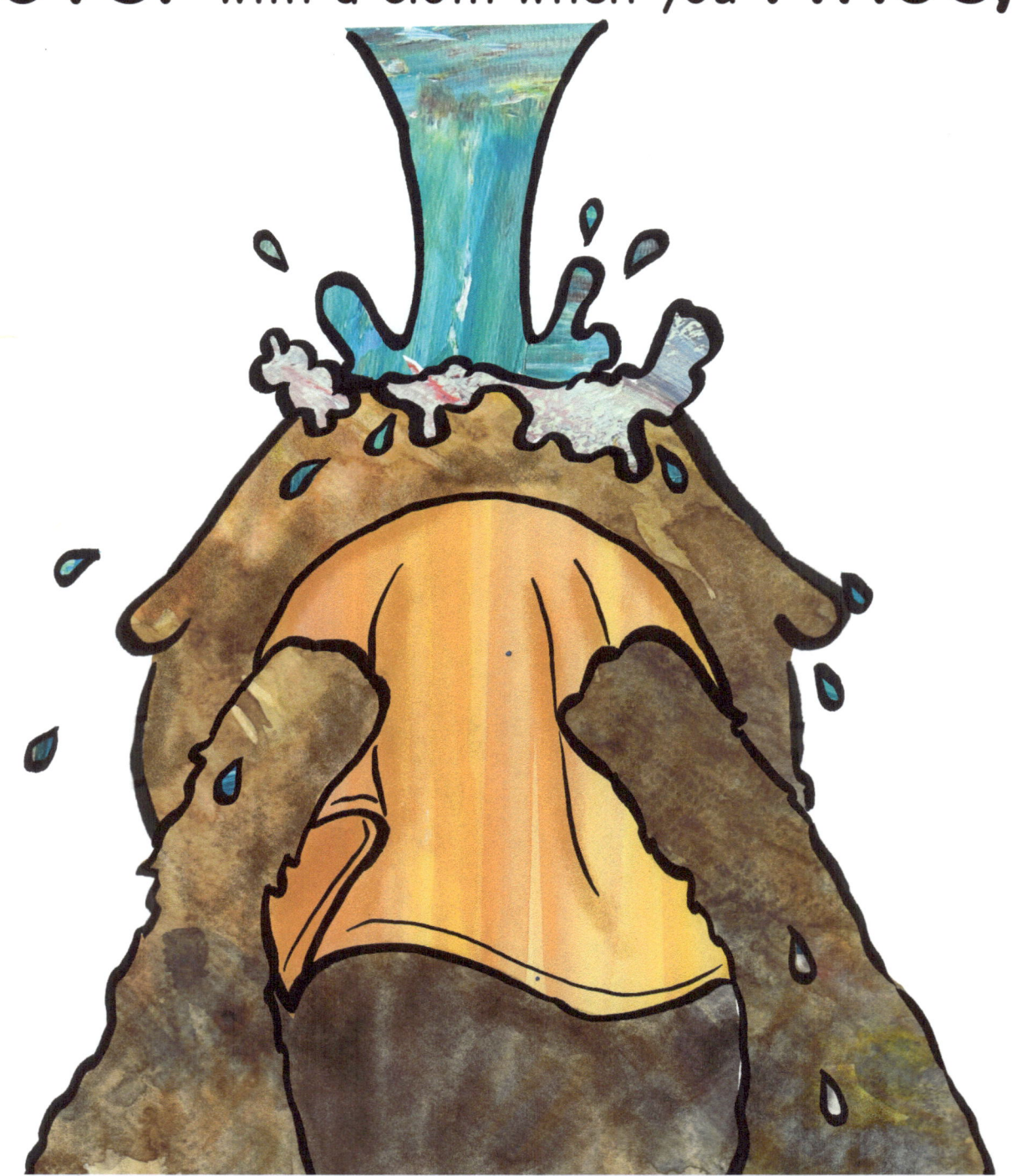

or wear a **visor** like a prince!

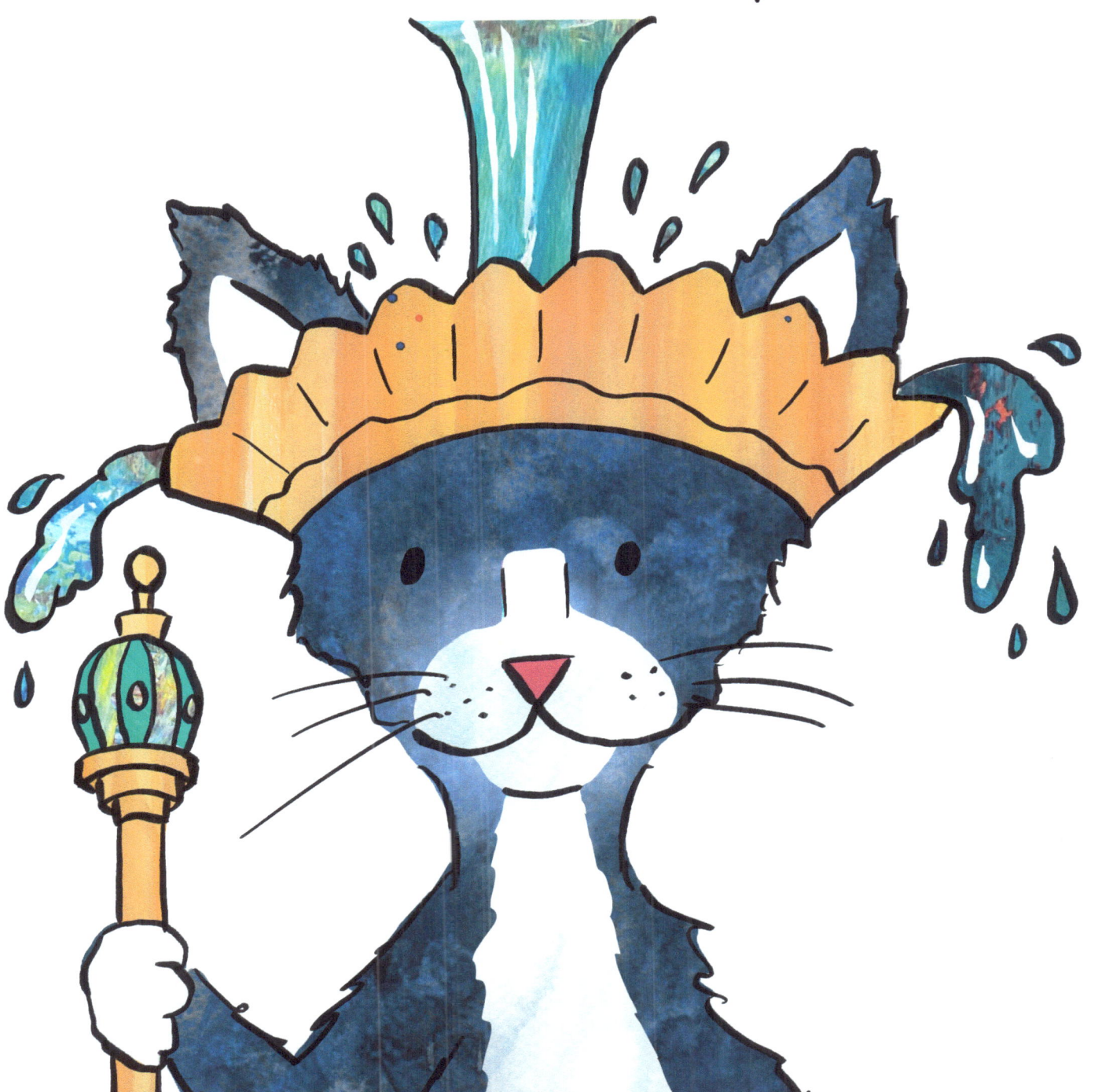

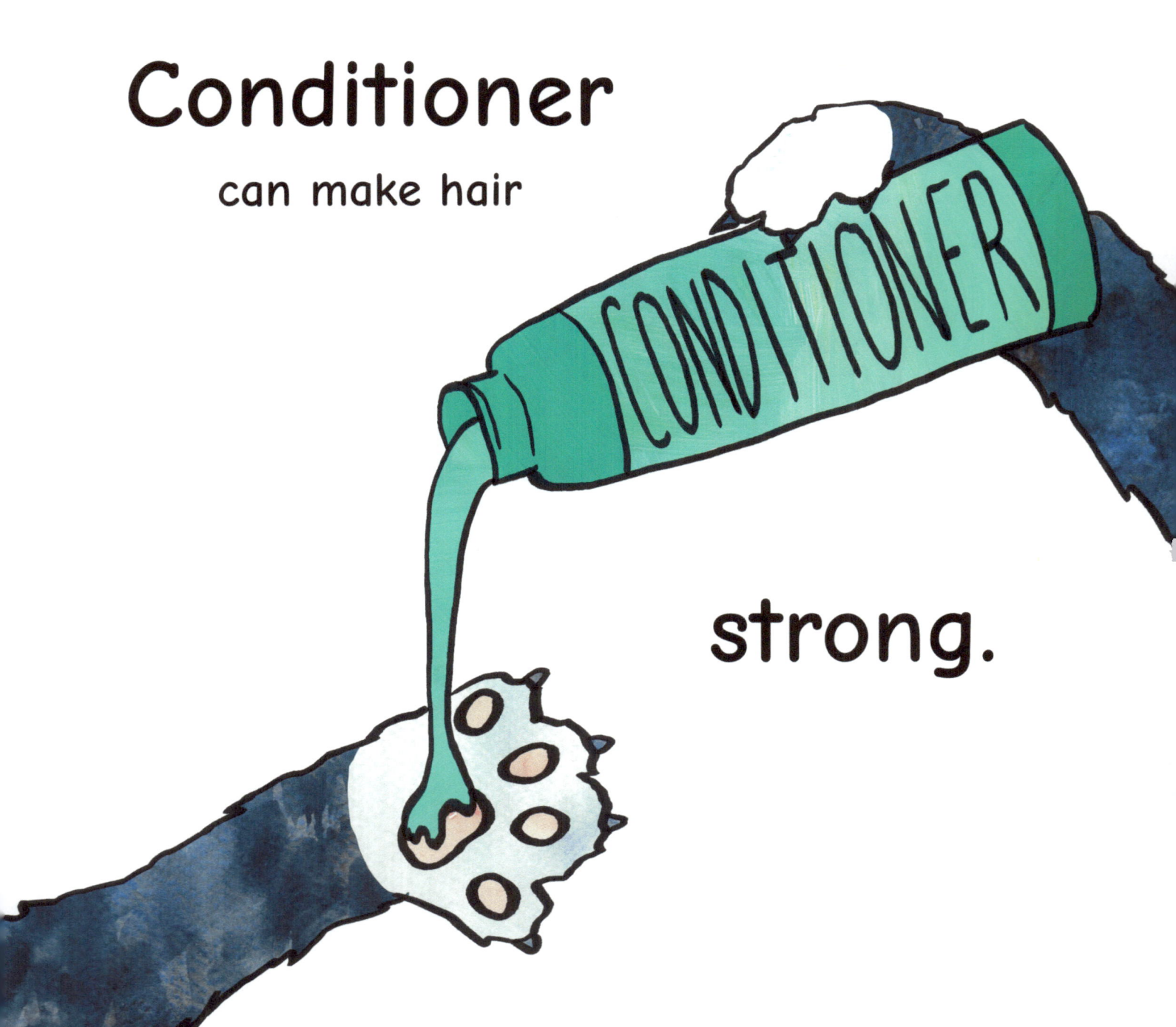

Conditioner
can make hair strong.

It goes

on hair

and stays there

long.

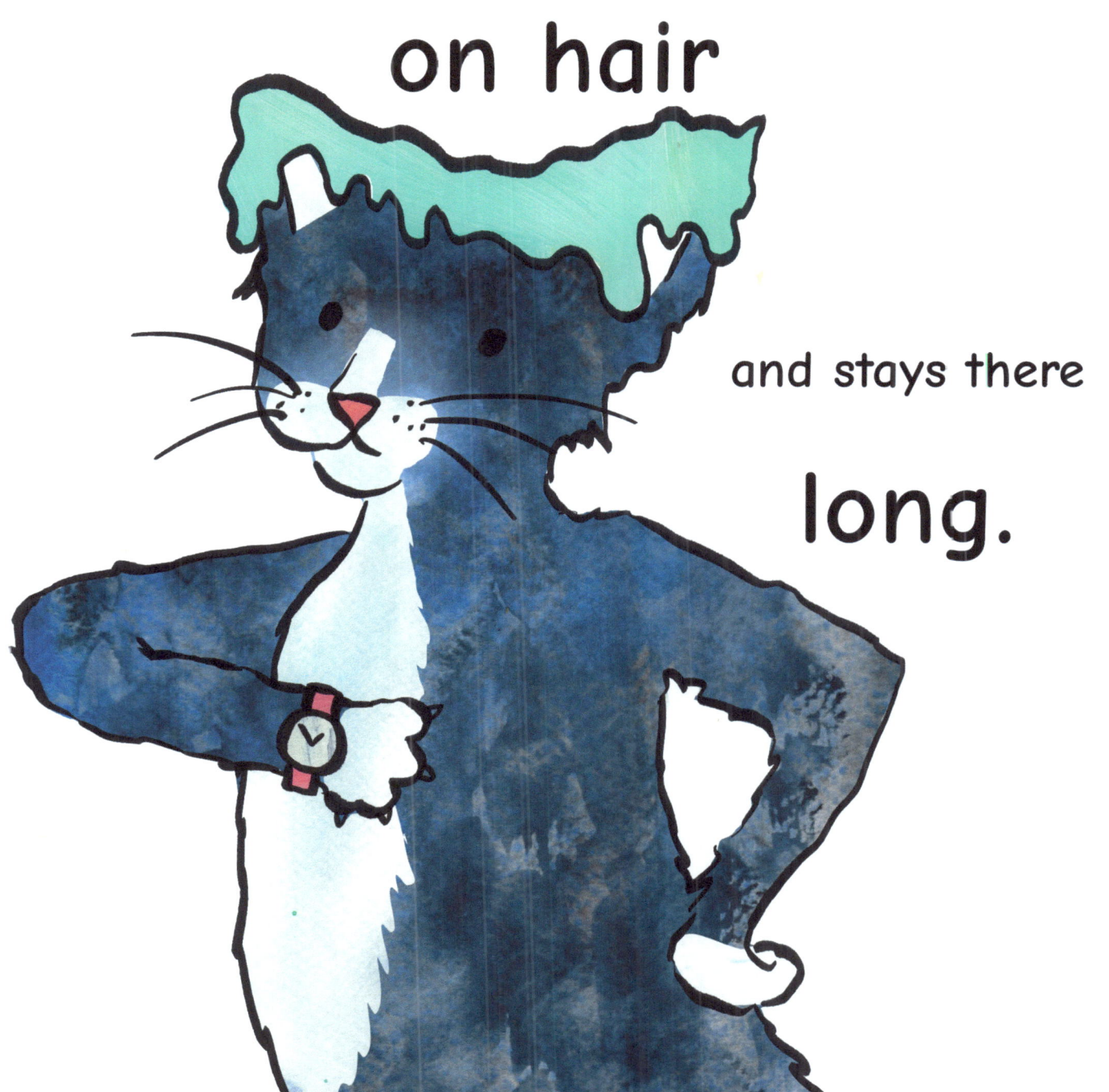

Soap all over and lightly scrub,

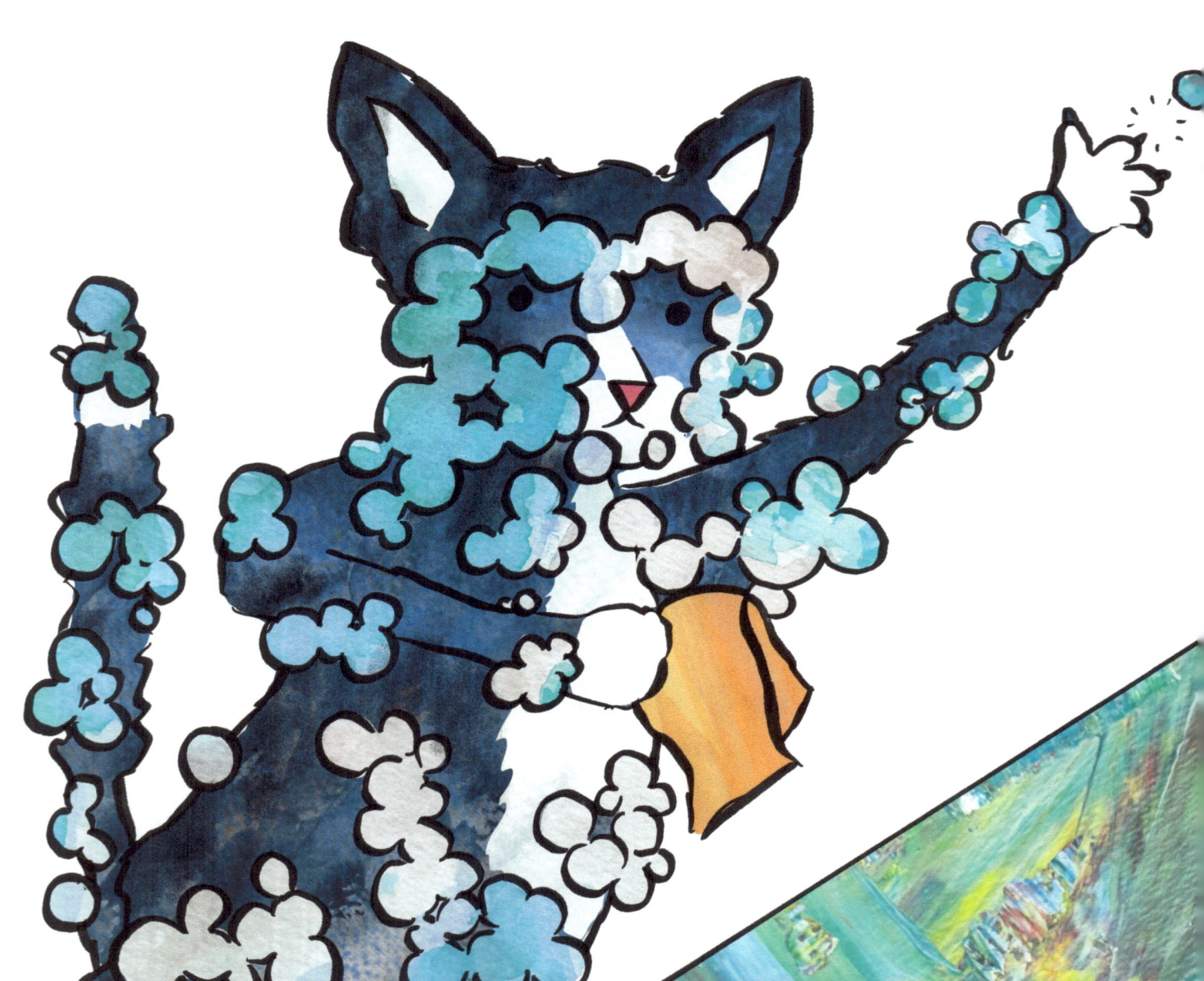

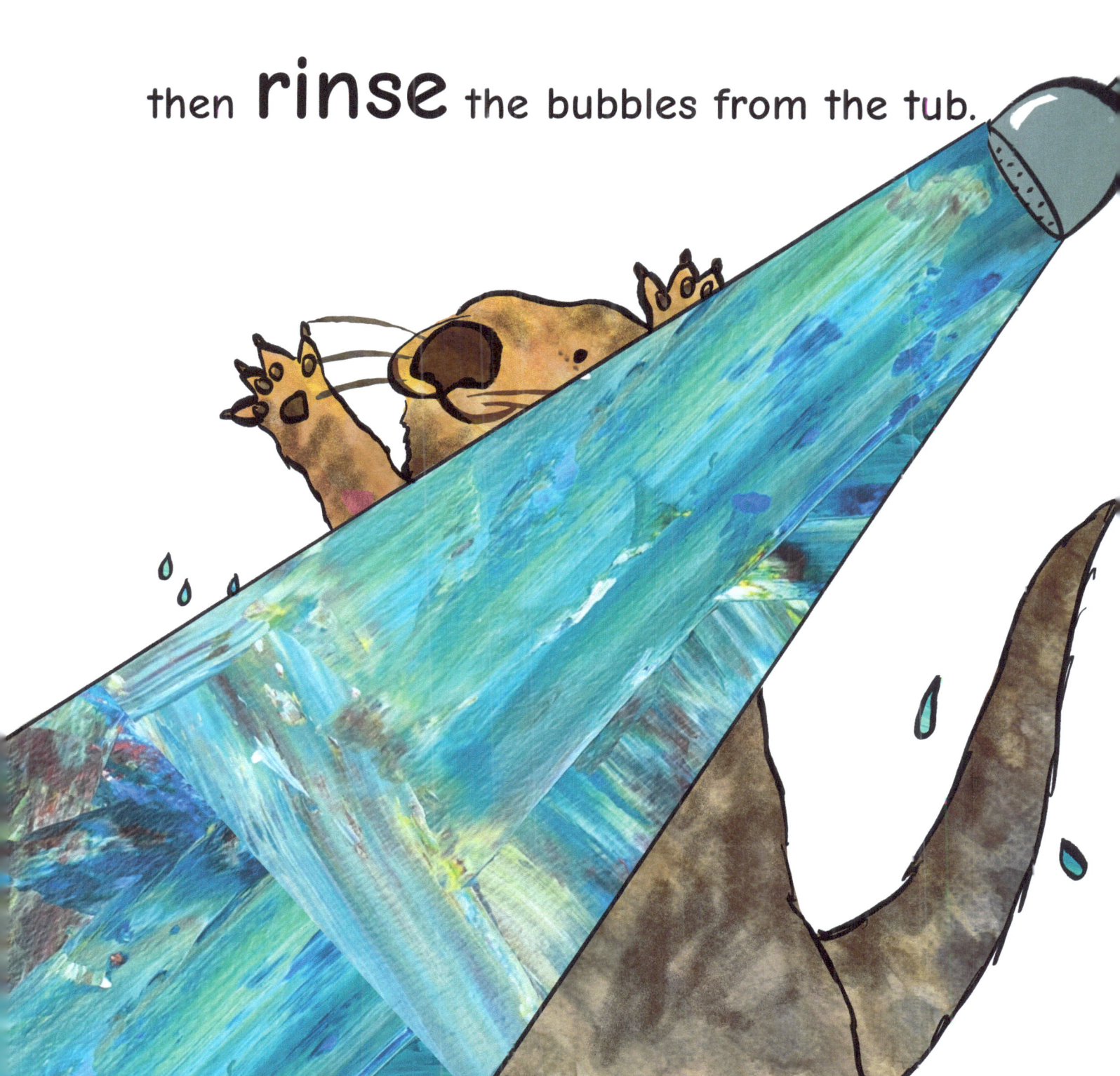
then rinse the bubbles from the tub.

Dry your body and dry your hair,

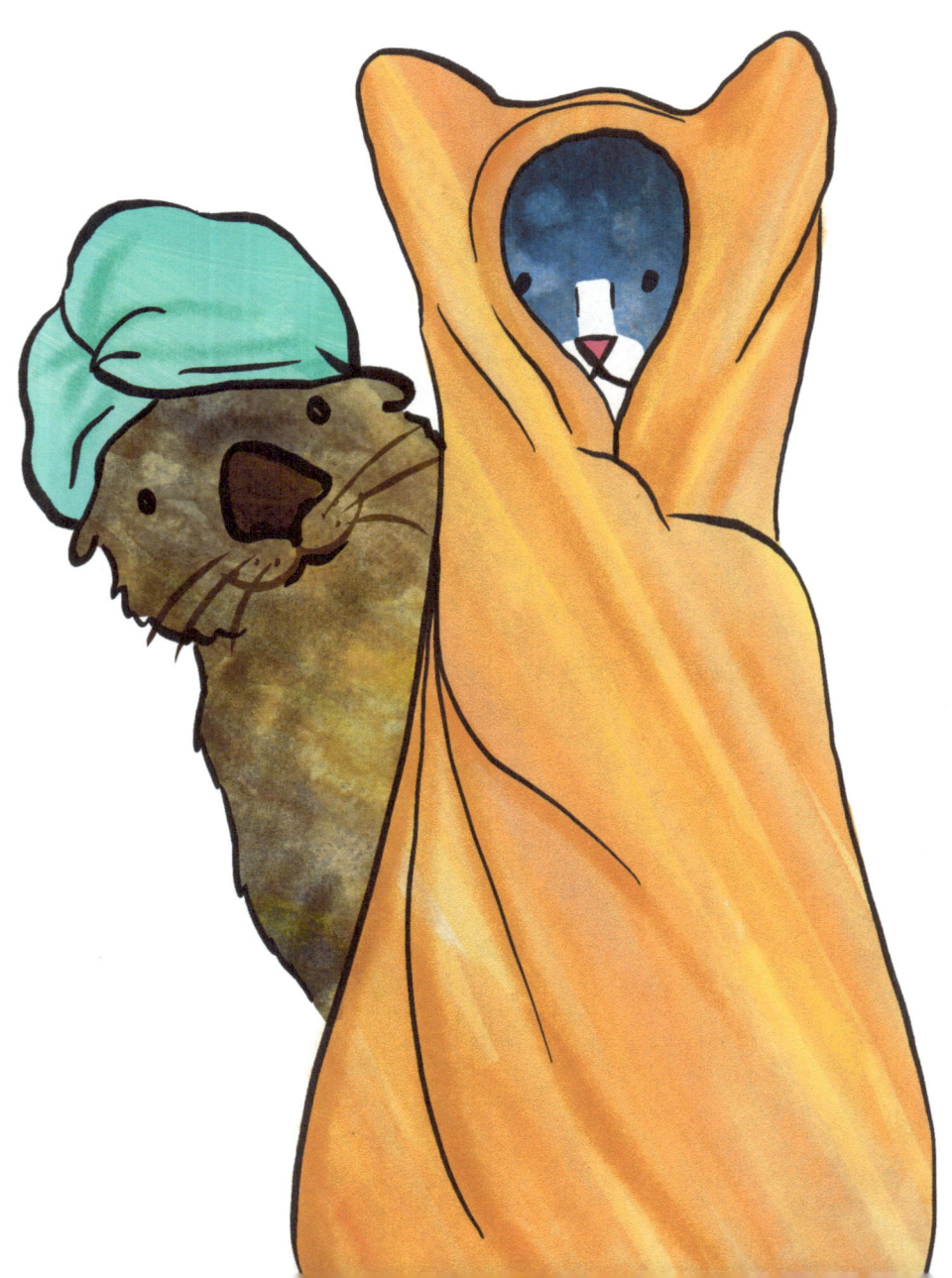

then go get some

clean clothes to wear.

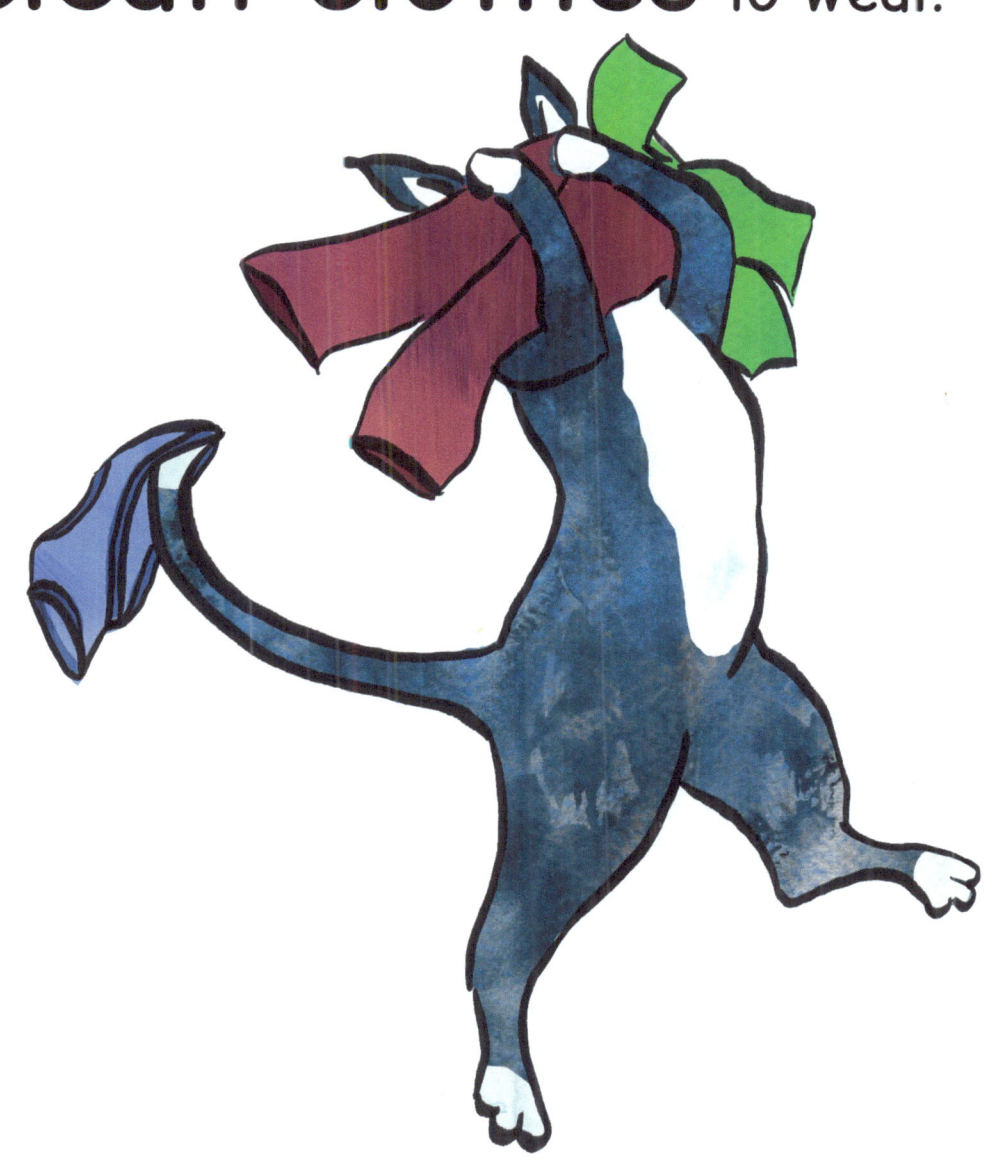

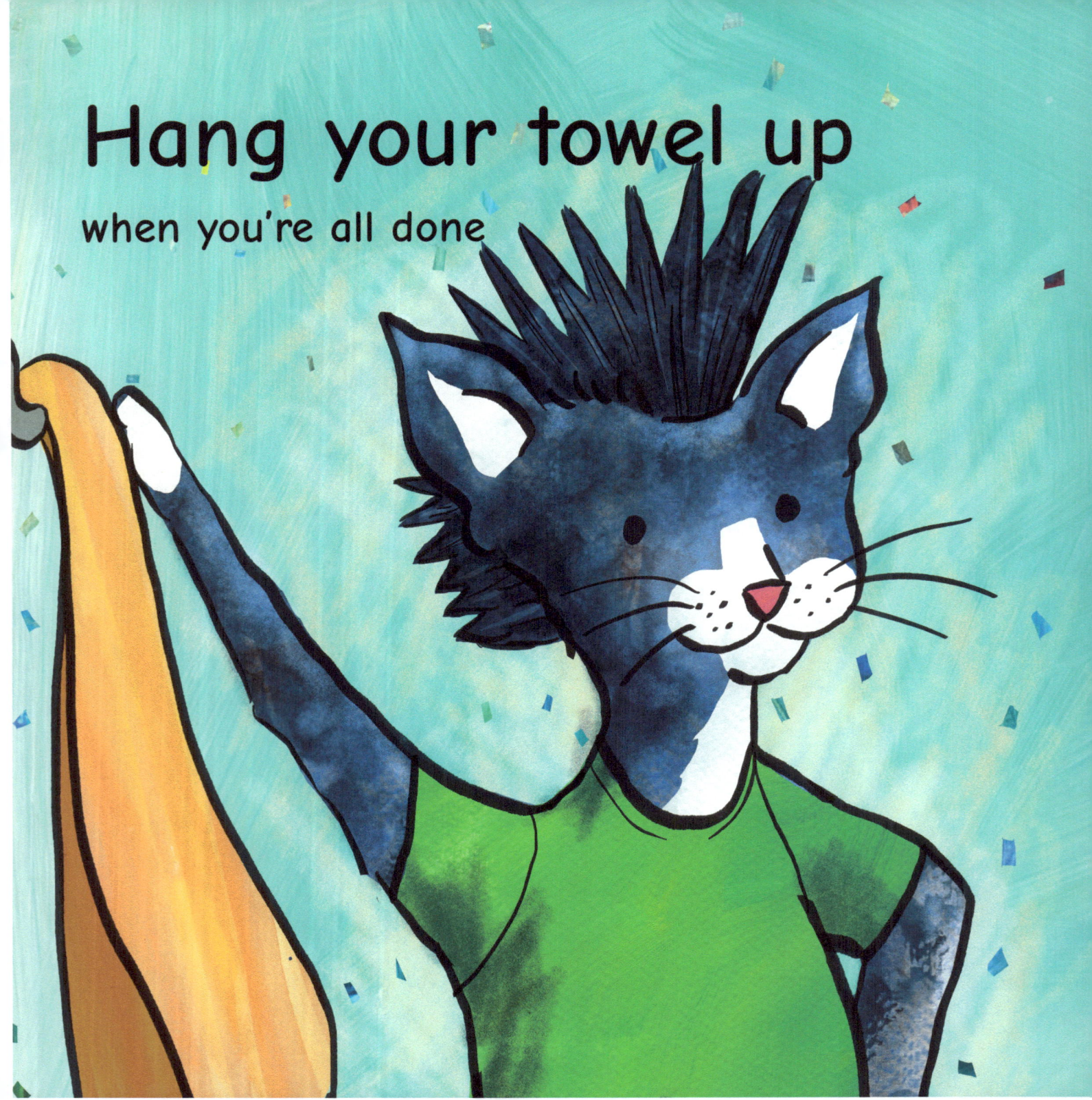

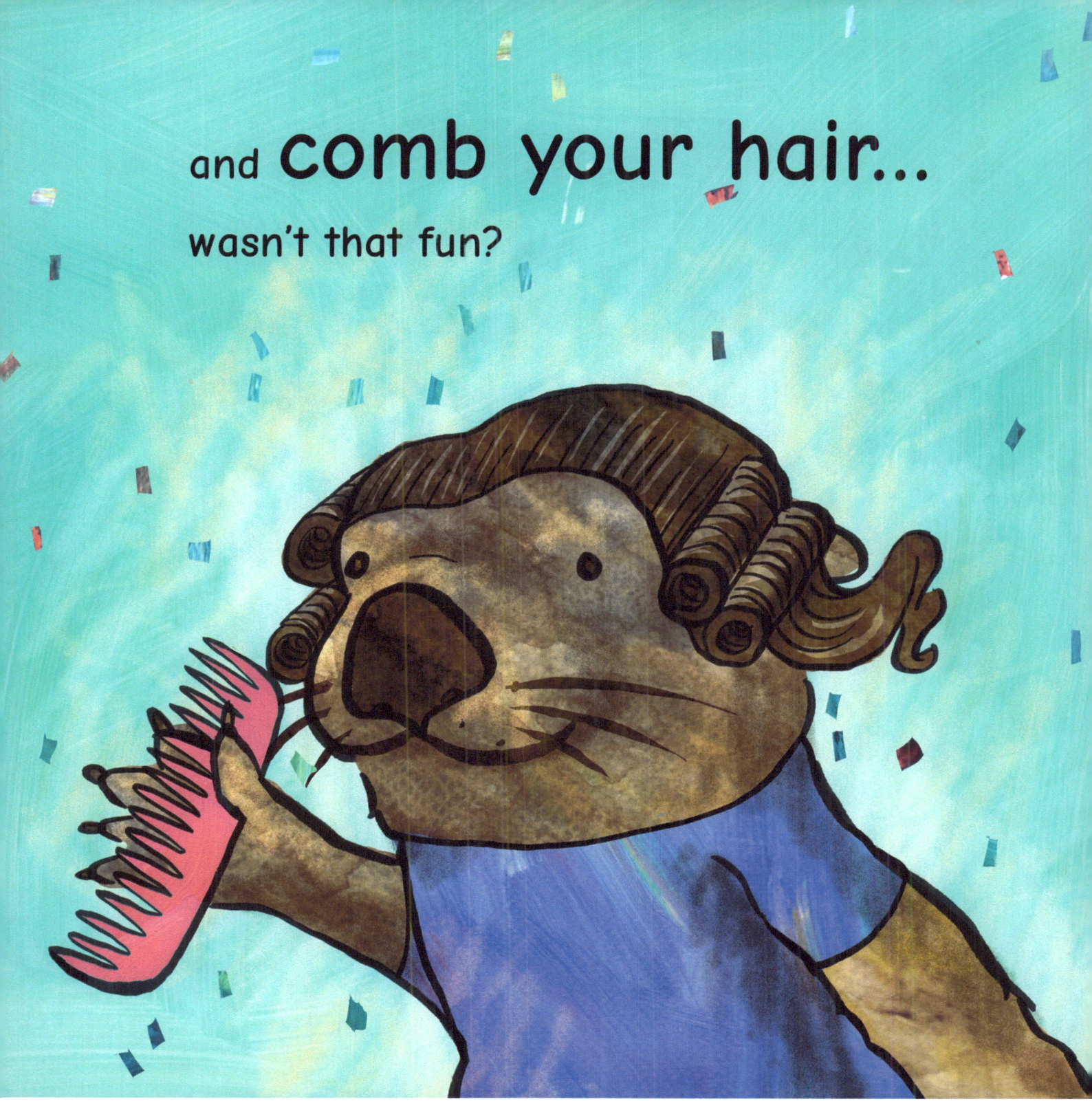

Thanks for reading!

If you enjoyed this book or found it helpful, please consider leaving a review or recommending it to a friend.

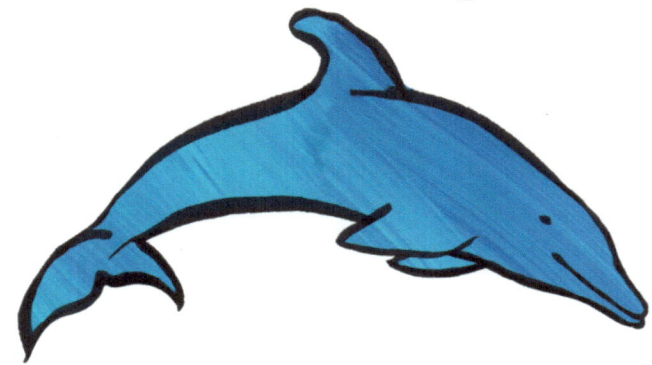

Stay up to date with the latest from Light Muse Studio, LLC by signing up for the newsletter on Substack and following me on socials.

Visit www.lightmusestudio.wixsite.com/home

for more information and extras.

The following pages are small versions of each illustrated step to copy or cut out and post as a visual reminder.

You could make this more interactive by cutting each image separately and having the child arrange the steps in the correct order with support.

Visit www.lightmusestudio.wixsite.com/home/stepsinrhymeprintables

if you need to print more copies for personal use.

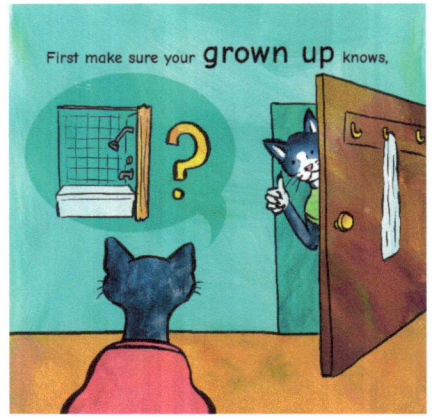
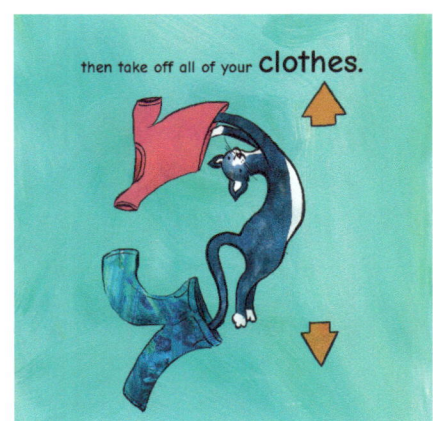
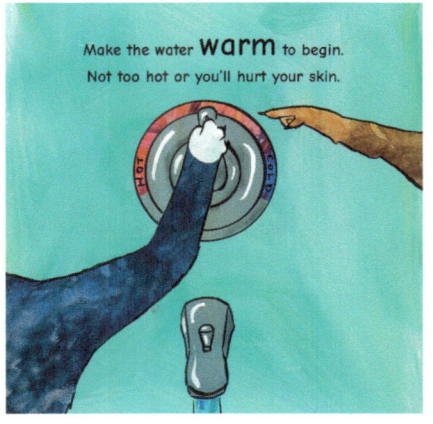
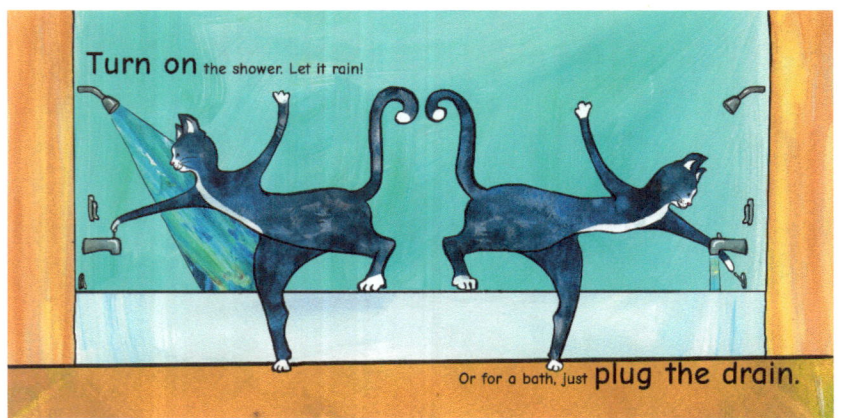
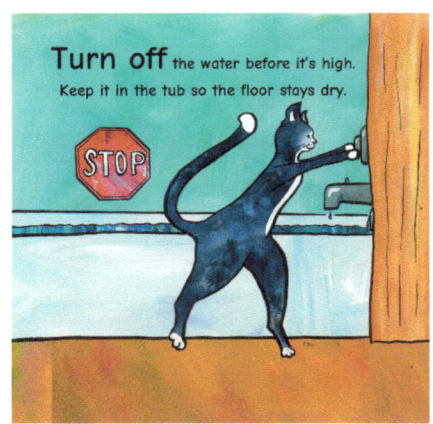
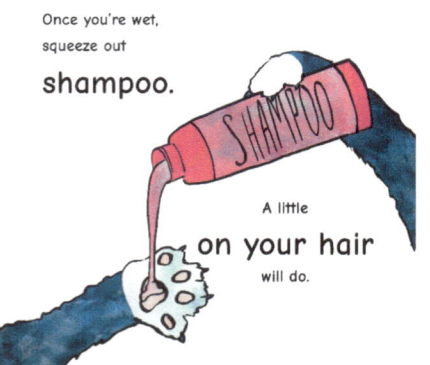
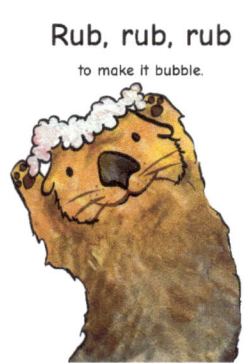
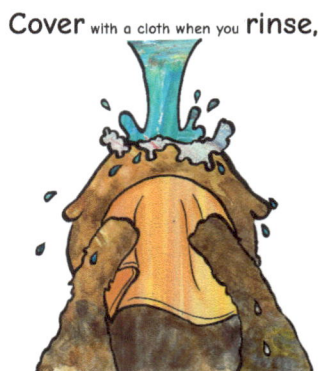

or wear a **visor** like a prince!

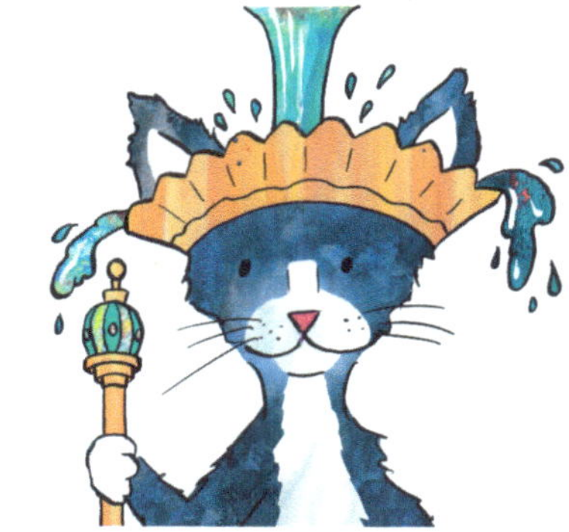

Conditioner can make hair **strong.**

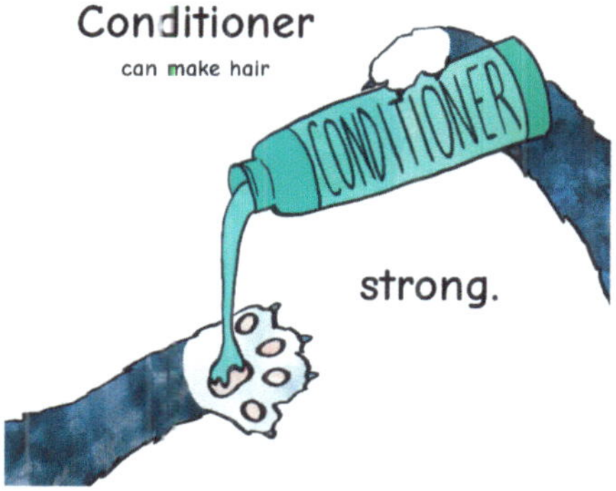

It goes **on hair** and stays there **long.**

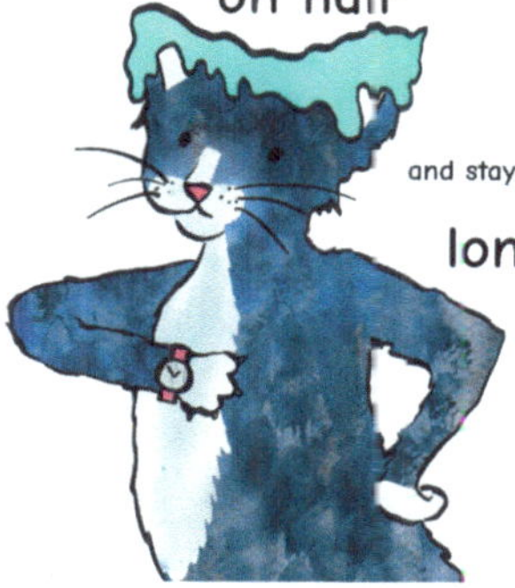

Soap all over and lightly scrub,

then **rinse** the bubbles from the tub.

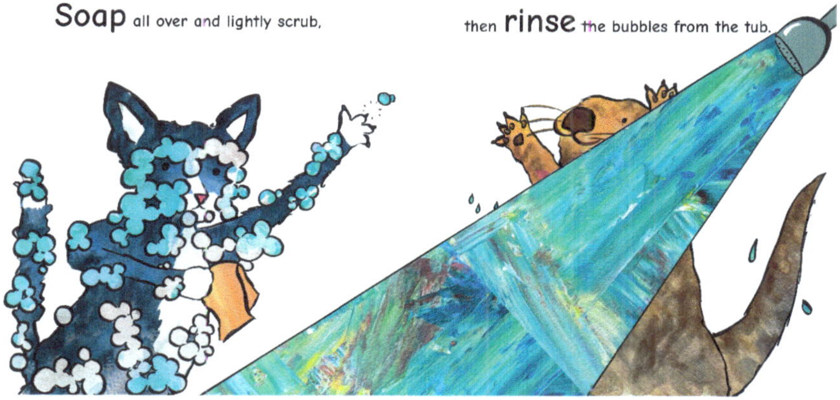

Dry your body and dry your hair,

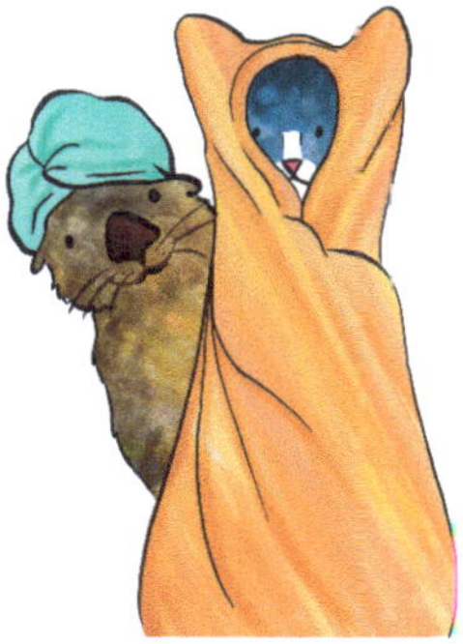

then go get some **clean clothes** to wear.

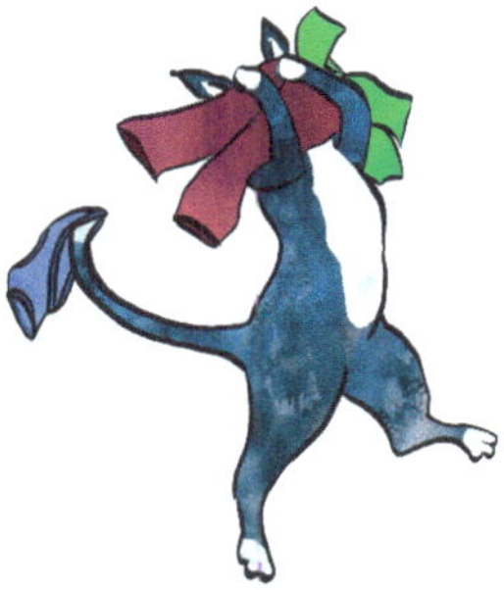

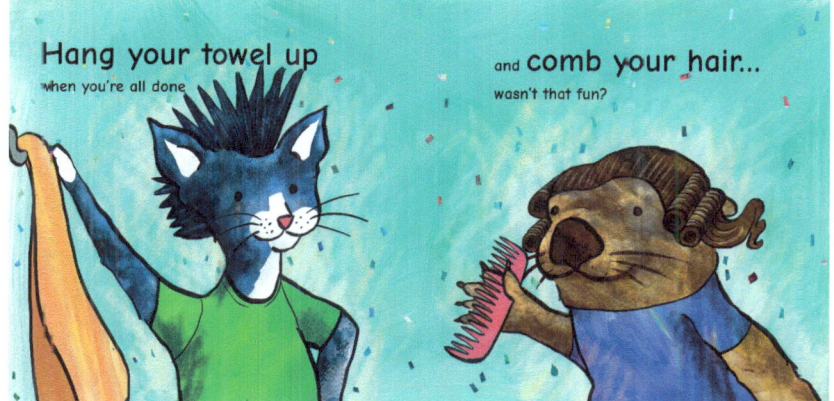

Hang your towel up when you're all done and **comb your hair...** wasn't that fun?

www.ingramcontent.com/pod-product-compliance
Lightning Source LLC
Chambersburg PA
CBHW061157030426
42337CB00002B/34